BREAST CANCER

BREAST CANCER

MY PERSONAL JOURNAL

VETAH OKUOMOSE

TATE PUBLISHING
AND ENTERPRISES, LLC

Published by Tate Publishing & Enterprises, LLC
127 E. Trade Center Terrace | Mustang, Oklahoma 73064 USA
1.888.361.9473 | www.tatepublishing.com

Tate Publishing is committed to excellence in the publishing industry. The company reflects the philosophy established by the founders, based on Psalm 68:11,
"The Lord gave the word and great was the company of those who published it."

Book design copyright © 2015 by Tate Publishing, LLC. All rights reserved.
Cover design by Bill Francis Peralta
Interior design by Mary Jean Archival
Cover picture courtesy of Dwi Sujadi

Published in the United States of America

ISBN: 978-1-68164-995-5
Biography & Autobiography / Personal Memoirs
15.08.11

Acknowledgments

To MY LORD, for His constant presence and guidance in my life.

To my beautiful family and my friends, thank you for being there for me!

To my supervisor at work, for your support and understanding, thank you

Special thanks to the infusion suite/radiation unit nurses and technicians at Mount Sinai St. Luke's and Mount Sinai Roosevelt Hospital for your cheerful faces and encouragement to each patient who walks through the door for treatment

To Dr. William Samson's office staff, such professional and great groups!

To the office staff at the Comprehensive Breast Center

To all my treating physicians and physician assistants, thank you!

INTRODUCTION

I BEGAN EXPERIENCING problems with my left breast in my late twenties. I felt a lump on the upper-outer quadrant, and I also had discharges from that same breast. The discharge was spontaneous and unilateral. At first, I was mortified, especially as I have had this irrational fear of cancer since nursing school. I began reading books about breast lumps and breast discharges. Although I was reading everything I could about breast diseases, I made sure I stuck to benign breast conditions. Breast cancer was out of the question. I did not want to know anything about signs and symptoms of breast cancer. When it comes to breast cancer, my attitude was like that of a frightened child with a blanket pulled over his/her head.

I was relieved when I read about a benign breast condition that exhibited the same symptoms as I had, so I self-diagnosed and convinced myself that it would resolve on its own. However, my leaky breast, as I called it, persisted and actually got worse. The discharge was becoming more persistent and frequent, and it was also embarrassing to say the least. My nightwear were stained from the discharge, and at one point, I started sleeping with a bra, just to avoid soaking my nightgown and my bed.

In early 2003, I finally mustered up the courage to tell my doctor about the lump and the leaky breast. He suggested I see a breast specialist, and he referred me to Dr. T. During my first consultation with Dr. T, he sent me to get a mammogram and a sonogram. On my follow-up visit with Doc T, he told me I had a very dense breast and that the palpable lump did not show up in either the mammogram or the sonogram. He recommended removing the lump and the ducts, which he said would fix the problem of the discharge.

First biopsy: I went in for the procedure accompanied by a friend; I was discharged home with pain meds. The day after the procedure, my breast felt like a rock! I went back to Dr. T about a week later, and he told me it was a good thing they removed the lump because it could have turned into something else because there were some atypical cells in the lump.

The final diagnosis read:

1. intraductal papilloma with atypia (0.5 cm.)
2. the rest of the breast shows fibrosis and florid ductal hyperplasia with focal atypia-microcalcification identified

I was so relieved! Dr. T recommended follow-up visits every six months and a yearly mammogram and sonogram due to the atypical cells. I went about my life as usual, and I was happy the problem of the leaky breast was finally solved.

Second biopsy: Needle localization with sonogram. My follow-up mammogram and sonogram, which were taken a year after the diagnosis, came back suspicious according to Dr. T; they found a lesion at the same location the lump was. He recommended a needle-localization biopsy, and I agreed to the procedure. The procedure was crude and horrible. First, the suspicious area was localized with the aid of a sonogram; then they inserted a long needle into my breast, with the long end of the needle sticking out; and then a cup was placed over the needle. There I was, looking so ridiculous, waiting in the hallway for my turn to go into the OR. It must have been four hours later before I was wheeled in. Although I was told I would not be under general anesthesia, it felt like it was afterward in the recovery room. I was very groggy, my breast was bleeding so much, and it took quite awhile to bring the bleeding under control.

I went back for the result and was told by Dr. T that it was benign.

The pathology report read:

1. Hyalinized intraductal papilloma with micro-calcifications (localized site)
2. Fibrocystic disease with florid ductal hyperplasia

Although I was happy about the result, I was a little concerned because it took some time for the wound to heal, and there was also an offensive odor each time the bandage was removed. It was tiresome going back and forth to Dr. T to have the wound dressed by him, but it finally healed up. I continued follow-up until February 2005.

After the second procedure, my breast was looking quite unattractive. Besides the scar, the breast was indented, the post-procedure hardening of the breast seemed to be there to stay, and the lumpiness grew worse; however, I was not troubled by all these. I convinced myself that it was due to the trauma from the two open biopsies. I also started experiencing this chronic pain on my upper left arm that I attributed to bursitis.

I went back a year later for a clinical exam and a follow-up mammogram and sonogram. The clinical exam and the sonogram were normal, but the mammogram showed abnormal microcalcification on the same left breast and at the same general location that had the history of the atypical cells. Dr. T recommended another biopsy, but at this point, I was tired of being poked and cut, so I asked him if we could just monitor it closely. He agreed. I continued with my regular follow-up with him.

November 2007

I WENT FOR my usual follow-up visit with Dr. T, the clinical exam was normal, and I had a mammogram and a sonogram done and was told that the previous finding in the mammogram was still there and biopsy was still recommended. I reluctantly agreed, but I requested to do it after the holidays.

Third biopsy. Stereotactic biopsy was performed on February 2008 by Dr. T and another doctor. I was made to lie facedown on an uncomfortable table with my breasts hanging down through a hole on the table. Underneath me was Dr. T and the other doctor, local anesthesia was administered to the breast, and I was required to lie still for about an hour or so while they simultaneously x-rayed the breast to visualize the location of the calcification. Next, a large gauge needle was introduced into the breast tissue to get some sample cells. It was so uncomfortable, and I was glad when it was over. The only good thing about this biopsy was that there was no cut.

I went for the results and was told by Doc T. that everything was fine.

The pathology report read:

1. Left breast, no calcification; stereotatic core biopsy: intraductal sclerosing papilloma. Fibrocystic change harboring micro-calcifications and including florid ductal hyperplasia, apocrine metaplasia, cysts, stromal fibrosis, sclerosing and blunt duct adenosis

2. Left breast calcifications; stereotactic core biopsy: Fibrocystic change harboring coarse calcifications and including florid and papillary ductal hyperplasia, stromal fibrosis, cysts and sclerosing adenosis

My breast, however, was getting increasingly disfigured, and the area of the biopsies became very lumpy and irregularly shaped. Over one-third of my breast from the top toward the axillar area became very lumpy and hardened. Although I was getting a little concerned about it, cancer was not even in my thought at that point. The three biopsies had been benign, and the clinical exams by Dr. T had been normal, and so far, he had not voiced any concerns. After all, he was the breast specialist, so I reassured myself that the reason for the lumpiness was due to the biopsies.

During the follow-up clinical exam with Dr. T, I voiced my concern about the lumpiness and hardening, and I even told him about the new lump I felt near the axilla (the Tail of Spence). He palpated me and told me he felt nothing abnormal.

I was sent for the usual mammogram and sonogram on August 2009. During the sonogram, I was paying particular attention to the technician's facial expression as she went over and over the lumpy area with the instrument. Surprisingly, both the sonogram and mammogram came back normal, and I remember breathing a sigh of relief when I read, "Congratulations, your recent mammogram and sonogram does not show any sign of cancer." Although I was relieved about the result, I just had this feeling that the result was too good to be true.

Shortly after that mammogram and sonogram, I started experiencing acute pain. I ignored the pain initially, attributing it to the compression from the mammogram, but I could not ignore the pain any longer. So about two months later, on October, I went back to Dr. T complaining of pain. He took one look at my file and stated, "You have a cyst." He inserted a needle into my breast near the areola, and he aspirated a syringe full of fluids. He told me to come back in three months if the pain persisted. He also ordered me to eliminate caffeine from my diet and take vitamin E.

I got a little relief from the pain but not completely, and after two weeks or so, the pain came back, and my breast was looking frightful; it was very asymmetric, lumpy, and hard. Although I was getting increasingly concerned over the way it looked, I kept reminding myself that cancer could not happen to me, therefore, it must be something acute, possibly from all the past trauma to the breast.

I went back to Dr. T five months later on March 2010, and he took one look at my breast, and he had this look of alarm on his face. Then I started to get worried! He seemed confused as to what to do next. First, he said, "Let's have an MRI based on your past history of atypical cells" (that was in 2003!), then he changed his mind, and said, "We should start out with a repeat sonogram." I went in for the sonogram.

I usually study the faces of the technicians as they perform the procedure, and most times, I am unable to read the expression on their faces because they usually wear a blank expression. They must have been trained to keep that blank expression on their faces! This time, this technician was looking alarmed as she went over my lumpy area with the instrument over and over again. Looking at her expressions made me afraid. I told myself, "I am doomed!" I went back to Dr. T for the verdict, and he told me I would need another biopsy because they found multiple nodules.

Sitting on the exam table and hearing Dr. T say I needed another biopsy was just too much for me. When was this ever going to end? For the first time, I was contemplating going to a real breast specialist; Dr. T was a general surgeon specializing in bariatric surgery! My friend Veronica had been trying to get me to change doctors for a while. She made some research and had given me a few phone numbers of some breast specialists previously, but being a creature of habit, I was not willing to start all over with a new doctor, so I decided to go ahead with the biopsy. I told Dr. T I needed to get an okay from my job and that I would call back to schedule the procedure.

I called back a week and a half later, and his secretary was surprised. She told me Dr. T wrote on my chart that I had refused biopsy! I was very upset. Why would he write that? For the first time in all these years I have been going to him, I requested a copy of the report of the sonogram. She faxed it to me, and to my chagrin, the report was mixed up. They were referring to the right breast as the diseased breast instead of the left. That was when I decided to see a breast specialist. I was mad at myself at this point. Why did I wait this long to find a real breast specialist?

I called Dr. T and left him a message, he later called me back that evening, and I told him in no uncertain terms that I was upset. "Why did you write in my chart that I refused biopsy?" I asked him, but he had no reasonable explanation to give. I also brought to his attention the mix-up on the sonogram report, which he told me he was aware of, and then I informed him I was going to a breast specialist, and he said, "Keep me posted."

I called the office of Dr. Sharon Rosenbaum Smith, a breast surgeon at the Comprehensive Breast Center at Mount Sinai St. Luke's and Mount Sinai Roosevelt. To make my appointment, I said to the lady on the other end, "I am not sure if the doctor will see me, because I do not have breast cancer." I made sure she knew that! "It is okay," she said. "She will see you." I suppose she must be used to potential patients who are in denial about their breast conditions!

I was very nervous about this appointment. At home, I would stand in front of the mirror looking at my breast and the ugly huge lump that was now covering more than one-third of my breast, and I'd tell myself it had to be the trauma from prior biopsies, it just has to be!

May 2010

THE DAY—WEDNESDAY—FINALLY CAME for my appointment. I prayed, "Lord, I can't afford to be sick!" I cried in my office because I was so scared! Then I picked up my Bible to read, and these words from Isaiah 41 seemed to leap off the pages at me: "Fear not, for I am with you; be not dismayed, for I am your God." I was so comforted by that scripture, it felt like I had God's arm around me!

A resident doctor took my history, and then Dr. Rosenbaum Smith came in and examined me. Her examinations were very thorough. (All these years Dr. T never examined me like that!) She was not happy at the size of my lump. She took one look at the films I brought from the previous institution and declared, "They are all mixed up, I will have to start all over." She informed me that I would need a new mammogram and sonogram. She also informed me she was going to do a fine needle aspiration (FNA) right then and there and that the result would be available in two hours. When I heard that, my body went cold out of fear. I started trembling all over; I was never as scared in all my life as I was that moment!

She used a portable sonogram machine to locate the area that she needed to get the cell sample, and then she inserted this frightening-looking syringe with a long needle into my breast, and in a few minutes it was over. I exhaled when she told me the result would not be available until the next day because it was already the end of the day. I was told to call back the next day for the result. The physician assistant took me downstairs to make the appointment for the mammogram and sonogram, which was on Friday.

May 20

I was holding my breath all day, too scared to call for the result; I was waiting for them to call me. As each hour went by with no phone call, I was a little less worried. I called in to my home phone to check for messages almost every 30 mins and sighs of relief when there were no messages.

The end of my work day came, and no message came from them, so I reasoned no news was good news! When I got home, however, I saw the doctor's number on my caller ID but no message. I thought to myself, *Okay, if it was significant news, they would have left a message.*

May 21

Friday at work, I waited again for the dreaded call, but there was none. Then it was time for me to go in to the city for the mamo and sono, which was in the same building as Dr. Rosenbaum Smith's office. I was driving into the city at about 3:30 p.m. when I got the call, It was, the physician assistant, asking me to come in to discuss the result of the FNA. I wanted to know right then and there; I couldn't wait the 15 minutes that it would take to drive there!

She told me she could not discuss the results over the phone. I knew right then it was not going to be good. "It is bad, isn't it?" I don't remember what she said, but I already knew.

On the phone with my friend, I told her I had cancer! She prayed for me as I raced to the doctor's office in total shock. I truly never thought I was going to hear that news. I honestly believed cancer is a disease others got, not me! None of my relatives close or distant had ever had cancer. I thought there must have been some mistake!

I don't know how I got to the doctor's office. I remember walking in a daze through the double doors that lead into the building. "It is cancer," said the doctor. I sat there, frozen. She told me there was not enough information about the cancer as the fine needle biopsy was a limited test, and that additional testing is needed to get more information about the cancer.

Not enough information! It is one thing to get this horrific news; it is another thing to get the news on a Friday evening and have to wait until after the weekend to learn my fate. *What type of cancer is it? What stage and has it spread?* All these questions would have to wait for the answer after the weekend. *Just shoot me now! How could I possibly make it through the weekend?* I burst into tears. Although she was encouraging, I couldn't hear anything else at that point.

I went downstairs for the scheduled mammogram and sonogram accompanied by the physician assistant; she was quite patient with me. As I sat there completing the forms before the mammogram, my tears were freely flowing. When she heard, my friend Veronica left work early to be with me. The mammogram technician was heaven-sent. She spoke such encouraging words to me, she told me not to fear, that God is in control of my life, she told me I was going to be okay, that the other day she had a hundred-year-old lady come in for a Mammogram, that she has had five breast cancers since she was fifty years old, and that she is still alive at one hundred. She even jokingly spoke of my future offspring as she put the shield to cover me waist down before the mammogram. Now that is faith! Her words brought me much comfort and hope.

May 22

I hardly slept all night; my stomach was trembling so hard, it was uncomfortable. All kinds of thoughts raced through my mind, thoughts of what ifs—what if it is in the advanced stage, what is going to happen to me? All these thoughts swirled around my head.

I got up very early in the morning, it must be adrenaline, and I got all my dirty clothes together went to the Laundromat with my roommate. Some friends came over later in the day with food and some comforting Christian music CDs. That was of much help to me. One particular CD I kept on all night songs such as "'Tis so Sweet to Trust in Jesus" and "In Christ Alone" (lyrics below) brought me such comfort and hope. I cried so much in my room, begging the Lord to help me.

In Christ Alone

In Christ alone my hope is found
He is my light, my strength, my song…
No guilt in life, no fear in death
This is the power of Christ in me
From life's first cry to final breath
Jesus commands my destiny
No power of hell, no scheme of man
Can ever pluck me from His hand
'Till He returns or calls me home
Here in the power of Christ I'll stand
(Newsboys)

'Tis So Sweet to Trust in Jesus

'Tis so sweet to trust in Jesus
Just to take Him at His word
Just to rest upon His promise
And to know thus saith the Lord

Jesus, Jesus how I trust Him
How I've proved Him o'er and o'er
Jesus, Jesus, precious Jesus
Oh for grace to trust Him more…
(Selah)

May 23

I went to church today. I told the choir administrator that I had cancer, and she announced to the choir, and they prayed for me. I just couldn't control my tears, I felt so embarrassed. I should have stayed home!

May 24

I had this vivid dream last night. In the dream, I was driving my car but was not inside the car. As I was steering the wheel, the car became increasingly difficult to manipulate. It started going so fast that it got out of my control, then the steering wheel broke apart from the car into a different direction, and the car raced away out of my sight. Then a man appeared. He picked up the steering wheel and then led me on a search for the car. To my amazement, we found the car right at the edge of this vast ocean. Just a few inches away from falling into the ocean, the man in my dream helped me put the car back together, and the foot mats and other accessories inside the car were washed. The last part of the dream was me inside the car driving away from this building with plants in the lobby area.

I woke up from the dream with such peace and assurance, I felt the Lord was showing me through the dream that the cancer in my body has not gotten too advanced and that He has control over how far it has gone!

Midmorning at work, I got a phone call from the doctor's office that caused me momentary distress. I was told I needed—in addition to the scheduled extensive biopsy on Tuesday—I would need to have an MRI and PET scan done! (PET scan is used to detect the spread of cancer to distant organs.) I could not imagine how I was going to get through the week with all these intimidating tests to look forward to. The date for the PET scan seemed like my doomsday!

4th Biopsy
May 25

I woke up with a feeling of trepidation. Thinking of the scheduled biopsy later on in the day, I could not fathom how I was going to make it through the week with the biopsy, MRI, and PET scan to look forward to. Many what ifs were going through my mind. What would the biopsy show, what will turn up in the MRI and PET scan? Although I thought back to the dream I had and got a little comfort from it, but still, it was a dream, and I must face the reality of the present.

This biopsy was different from the previous ones done by Dr. T; this was done by the physician in the diagnostic office, not in the operating room. My breast was scrubbed and prepped by the technician assisting the radiologist, then the radiologist used the transducer to go over my breast, and guided by the sonogram, he inserted this intimidating-looking needle into my breast to get the tissue needed. Originally, he was to biopsy three locations, but then a call came that he should not bother to cover all the areas. That got me worried because I realized that the decision was based on the report of the mammogram and sonogram that was done on last Friday. I cried a little as I lay there.

May 26

Thursday Morning: I had a terrible night. So worried about the PET scan scheduled for Friday, I had a rough day. Thoughts of the biopsy result also caused me major anxiety. I remember just talking with the Lord quietly on my way home. *Lord I need a reassuring word to get me through Friday.*

I got home with absolutely no appetite or the desire to make dinner, then I got a call from the physician assistant, regarding the biopsy result. She told me the right breast was fine, and the cancer on the left breast was ductal carcinoma in situ (DCIS), slow growing, which means that the probability of it invading distant organs are slim. Although that initial report was not completely accurate, but that was all I needed to hear at the moment. *Thank you, Lord, you are good to me!* My appetite came back, and I had a good dinner.

You hear me, you answer
You rescued me, oh, Lord, you care.
Feeling overwhelmed,
It seems there is no end in sight.
I whispered a prayer,
If only He hears me,
If only He would answer,
If only He would rescue me,
When I least expected there you were.
You parted the dark clouds,
You moved the mountain.
Every prayer every tear,
Every cry of my heart.
Every silent prayer
You heard
Oh, Lord, you hear me!

Prior to the cancer diagnosis, I had stayed completely away from reading about breast cancer. But after the diagnosis, I just couldn't read enough about it. I devoured *Dr. Susan Love's Breast Book*. The book has such wealth of information regarding breast pathologies and especially breast cancer. I read about diagnostic tests, mastectomy, breast reconstruction, chemotherapy, and radiation. I also went online to learn about the various kinds of breast cancer, diagnostic testing and implications, various treatments options, etc. I wish I had read all these earlier!

MRI and PET scan
May 28

Today, I had the MRI and PET scan. My friend Onie took time off her busy practice to come with me for moral support. I am amazed at the peace in my heart! MRI was not so bad; I had my veins injected with contrast dye, then was made to lay still on my stomach with my breast hanging through an opening. I was given ear plug because inside the MRI was very noisy as the films were being taken, it took about forty-five minutes, I had such peace, I was almost falling asleep by the end of the procedure!

PET scan also was not so bad, except for the white chalky stuff I had to drink. I thought I would not see the end of it! Then a contrast dye was injected into my veins. I was made to lie on this uncomfortable table my head stabilized on each side, and then they told me to keep still, while the technician quickly left the room and the heavy metal door closed behind him. The intimidating-looking machine swirling around, as the table I was laying on slowing passes through from head to toe.

It is end of the week! I have never in all my life been poked and pulled like I have been this whole week. I am so thankful to the doctor and her assistant for taking such good care of me; all my appointments were made for me, I did not have to call or try to figure out insurance issues. It would have been so overwhelming if I had to. Now, the entire tests are done, I will have to wait for my verdict! I should be worried, but I am not. I have this incredible peace! These words from the bible kept me in check: "Do not worry about tomorrow…Be still and know that I am God" (Psalm 46:10).

Saturday. Woke up with no anxiety, went shopping with some friends, bought a few knickknacks for the living room, and got some clothes on sale.

May 31

As I sit this morning apprehensive of what the week will bring, I got thinking about what it is I am learning through all these. It is not about the severity of cancer or the baffling way this cancer seem to have presented itself, what I am learning most of all is the character of the Lord. I am learning of God's compassion toward me, His tenderness, and that he would humble himself to see my situation, feel my pain, sorrows and fears and address it. That God would anticipate my fears and anxieties and speak to me before it happens. *Oh, Father, yes, tomorrow is a mystery to me, but you know what it holds and have already made provision for it. Lord, I believe, help my unbelief!*

3

June 1

I MET WITH Dr. Rosenbaum Smith to learn my fate. The MRI confirmed the cancer on the left breast, and the mass was very big about eight centimeters! How could Dr. T have missed that! Right breast suspicious lesion was detected, and I will have to undergo further biopsy on the right breast. I was not too happy about that. PET scan result. Although there were some cells detected in my auxiliary lymph node, there are no distant metastasis! She told me, however, that due to the size of the mass, I would have to get a mastectomy—double, if the right breast shows any cancer! *Oh, Father, please let me keep my right breast!*

The doctor stated that there is a high probability that there is an invasive cancer in my breast contrary to the first pathology report, which says it is *DCIS* [DCIS is a stage 0 cancer that has not broken out of the duct]. "The fact that the PET scan is showing node involvement, there must be an invasive cancer in there," she said.

June 3

I met with Dr. William Samson plastic and reconstructive surgeon and his assistant Samantha Vogel, RPA, at Mount Sinai St. Luke's and Mount Sinai Roosevelt today—accompanied by my friend Ufuoma, an OR nurse; I figure she can ask the doctor some questions that I may miss. They were very reassuring. After examining me, he told me I did not have enough fat in my body (stomach) to do reconstruction; I would have to get an implant. I was disappointed because I was hoping to use my own tissue for the reconstruction, and for once, I envied those who were paunch-bellied! He explained the procedure to me after the mastectomy, which involved removing all the breast tissues and some muscles. The skin is spared, and then he is going to place a tissue expander inside and sew me back up. After a couple of weeks, they are going to inflate the expander with saline for a couple of weeks to stretch the skin, and after the skin is stretched to the desired size, he will go back in and remove the expander, then replacing it with a permanent saline or silicone implant. I decided on the saline implant.

June 4

I told my coworkers today about my cancer diagnosis, they were all so kind and encouraging.

June 8

The surgery was scheduled for the 16th. I just wanted to get the cancer out of me! I started grieving the loss of my breast even before the surgery. I would stand in front of the mirror looking at both breasts with such a sense of sadness and disbelief. "I can't believe I will be losing my breast in a week's time!" I kept saying sadly to myself, staring at both breasts. Even with the lumpiness and disfigurement, they looked so beautiful to me. "Oh, that I may keep one! Please let the right breast be okay!" I whispered a prayer.

June 10

The right breast stereotactic biopsy was particularly difficult today. Lying on my stomach with my breast hanging down through the opening, the technician was so rough pulling and tugging at my breast. She seem to have had some difficulty positioning the breast. I was impatient with her at one point because she seemed insensitive. I was instructed to keep still in that uncomfortable position for over an hour. The radiologist seems to also have difficulty locating the area to be biopsied; I was getting very frustrated and wept some. Finally, it was over, and the specimen was sent to the lab. I prayed it comes back benign!

Had some good news when I got home, the BRCA 1 and BRCA 2 tests came back negative (gene tests done to detect susceptibility to both breast and ovarian cancer). Oh yes, I forgot to mention earlier that I was seen by a genetic specialist after my diagnosis, who went down my family tree to determine if I had a family history of cancer, and then blood was drawn to determine if I had a gene that mutates. I learned something new from that meeting, that only 10–15% of all cancer happens in people with family history; the vast majority are seen in people without any family history of the disease.

June 11

I was a little anxious about the oncoming surgery. I prayed and trusted the outcome to the Lord. Great news, the right breast biopsy came back normal, I can keep my right breast!

June 13

A friend asked me the other day if I wasn't angry at God for my situation. I told her no, not sure if she believed me or not. I got thinking afterward about her question. The amazing thing is that since the whole ordeal with the diagnosis and the various tests I had to undergo, anger and questioning has not even crossed my mind! I do not feel that God has been unfair to me—in fact, all I feel is gratitude toward God for his love, for His comfort, and for allaying my fears. Yes, circumstances right now may seem against all that I desire, yet I do not feel angry. I know, for sure, I am not in denial.

June 15

I got a surprise call from one of my church leader today, very encouraging, and he prayed for me.

In just a few hours, I would be in the operating table having one breast removed and entering a new phase in my life! I am amazed at this peace in my heart and around me. This must be what it feels like when God is holding your hands—such a quite peace, no anxiety, no fear, just this peace!

June 16

Surgery day. Still have this incredible peace this morning. My brother flew in last night to be with me. I know he is very worried about me; I can see it in his face, though he is not saying much. It hurts me to see him looking so sad and anxious. I just wanted to make him see that I am going to be okay. Got through the preliminaries. The surgical gown was so huge, it swallowed me up, made me feel so ugly! A friend from church Willie, Veronica, and my brother kept me company as I waited to be called into the OR. Dr. Samson the plastic surgeon came to mark me up for the reconstruction phase of the surgery; he was like a skilled artist with his marker as he carefully marks the area around my breast.

Inside the operating room, the breast surgeon was so kind to me. She stood with me making small talk before the anesthesia kicked in. The last thing I remembered before going under was me crying silently and Dr. Rosenbaum Smith taking my hand as she consoled me.

I woke up in the recovery room hearing Dwi's voice, saying, "Don't cry."

Up in my room a few hours after the surgery, I had a full room! My aunt Eki (flew in from Atlanta), uncle Ben and aunt Christy from new Jersey, my brother, and my friends from church were all with me. I was up in bed in no time talking and laughing with them. They were all amazed at how quick I recovered from the anesthesia. I had something to eat later in the evening, and surprisingly, I was in good spirit!

June 17

The doctor came to see me the morning after accompanied by an intern. She confirmed what she had suspected before. There were two types of cancer found: a 5-cm invasive cancer and an 8-cm DCIS! In addition, there were three lymph nodes involved. I have been so baffled by this whole ordeal, an 8-cm DCIS and a 5-cm invasive cancer does not grow overnight. How was this possible considering I was closely followed by Dr. T for 7 years? I was not happy. A little while later, Dr. Samson came. He inspected the site (the tissue expander made me look like I still have a breast); the drain attached had some fluids collecting. He said everything looked good and that I should be discharged later in the day!

June 18

Home sweet home. It was good to sleep on my own bed again although did not get much sleep due to pain and fear of dislodging the drain. I was only allowed to sleep on my back, very uncomfortable as I usually sleep on my side and my stomach, difficult to find a comfortable position. The surgical bra also was very uncomfortable. Looking forward to ditching it for sports bra, hope I can do that next week! Everyone is amazed at my progress, and I am amazed at my peace.

June 19

My poor roommate seem to be taking this whole thing harder than I am. She is looking so stressed, quiet understandable as two of her coworkers came down with the dreadful disease, and one has already succumbed to the disease not so long ago. She does not understand how I can be so calm. She said to me the other day, "You don't always have to be strong." But I am not strong! If only she understands that I am not trying to put on a brave front; I am the most cowardly human on the face of this earth if left to my devices. But having God as my father, I have this strength and courage that is not of me. If only my walls could talk, they would tell her of my desperate cry to the Lord time and time again. They would tell of the fears that threatened to paralyze me when I dwell on the what ifs, they would tell of a child crawling into the arms of her father in total weakness, and they would also tell of the strength that comes suddenly from believing when God speaks. No, I am not strong at all—in fact, I am surprised at my peace, at this strength, only God could do this!

June 22

At Dr. Samson's today, the drain was removed, and I am free at last! He said the surgical site looked good.

June 28

Follow-up visit with Dr. Rosenbaum Smith day. Final diagnosis: invasive ductal carcinoma (5 cm–stage 2) with lymph node involvement and ductal carcinoma in situ (DCIS 8 cm). She told me the invasive component of the cancer was the aggressive type, HER2 positive, and I would need aggressive-preventative treatment with chemo and radiation. She gave me a referral to the oncologist, then the reality of facing chemo hit me hard, and I cried my eyes out.

Lord I need you!

I went over to see Dr. Anupama Goel, oncologist at Mount Sinai St. Luke's and Mount Sinai Roosevelt, who mapped out the medication regimen for me: I will be taking Carboplatin, Taxotere, and Herceptin, every three weeks for six circles, then after the sixth circle, I will continue on the Herceptin alone for a year.

She told me some of the side effects includes, but not limited to, hair loss, immediate menopause, in some cases cardiac damage, and low white count and red count to name a few!

She told me I would need a MUGA scan before the start of chemo. *What in the world is that?* She also advised me to get a port put in to minimize vein damage from the chemo. *A port! Wow, now, I am really going to look sick!* I thought to myself. It seemed like she read my mind. She offered to take me to the infusion suite to see what the port site looked like on the patients. The infusion suite was a large room with lodging chairs and TVs on each corner, curtain partitions for privacy, and IV poles with medications infusing into the patients. The port is placed under the skin (upper chest area) surgically, only a bump is visible to the eye.

As I was going into the elevator after my meeting with Dr. Goel, this bubbly elderly lady walked in with me. She asked me, "Are you getting a port?" She proceeded to show me hers and tell me she has had it for 9 years! That simple encounter encouraged me so much; it alleviated my anxiety about getting one put in.

I got home feeling so exhausted and overwhelmed—what a day! So much information to process. Sad about the prospect of losing my hair and going into menopause, I was hoping to have at least one child when my husband finally shows up! It is bad enough my biological clock is ticking away; this medication is just going to stop the clock completely! Hair loss. I couldn't find a husband with a head full of hair, how much more with no hair at all!

Lord, please give me a miracle, minimize the side effects, no permanent menopause, no infertility, no cardiac damage, and no infections.

4

July 1

MULTI GATED ACQUISITION heart scan (MUGA scan): First, the technician drew my blood; my right arm have been so abused (since blood can only be drawn from my right arm), it took the technician a while to get sufficient blood from me. After the blood was drawn in a test tube, it is then placed in some radioactive container to be "cooked" for a few minutes, and then that same blood, which I presume is now radioactive, is injected back into my veins. Then I was made to lie on this uncomfortable exam table hooked up to a heart monitor with EKG leads placed on me, then this intimidating machine with a camera on it, looming over my chest, the picture of my heart function is then visualized on the computer. The scan is used to test the strength of the heart valve before chemo therapy starts and, I was told, would need to continue with the scan periodically during the course of the therapy because of the damaging effect of one of the chemo medications on the heart muscle.

It took about an hour. The procedure was painless except for the needlestick, of course. I do not remember any special instructions after the test.

July 3

Went shopping for wigs today, had fun with my friends trying on various lengths and texture of wigs.

July 5

I am a little worried today about the chemo and how I will react to it. I have come to terms with the hair loss since I am told it will grow back. I just do not want to be incapacitated by the side effects of the meds. Will I be able to go to work? I need to work! Will I be made permanently sterile? What about my organs? Can my heart, liver, kidney, and GI handle the assault? *Oh, Lord, I bring all my fears to you, I pray for a miracle, quiet my fears in Christ's name. Amen.*

He guards all his bones not one of them is broken.

—Psalm 34:20

Port Catheter Insertion
July 8

> He will shield you with his wings. He will
> shelter you with his feathers. His faithful
> promises are your armor and protection.
>
> —Psalm 91:4

Today, I am encouraged by that scripture. As I walk through the valleys of the unknown, I have peace in my heart knowing God has control over the outcome. I believe the outcome of all these will be good.

I got to the interventional radiology unit by 10:30 a.m., accompanied by my friend Janice. Nothing by mouth after midnight, I waited for so long to be called. Could not handle the wait any longer and needed to take my pre-chemo medications (starting chemo next day, was instructed to take some meds a day before the start of chemo), so I took a sip of hot chocolate to take my meds. I was called in shortly after that! The nurse made such a big deal about the hot cocoa. She informed me I will not be getting any sedation for the procedure due to risk of aspiration. I think she was making a mountain out of a mole hill. She told me I will only be getting pain medication and local anesthesia. Anyway, I got to the room, I was draped on the exam table. The doctor was not very personable, he had some students watching the procedure, and he was busy teaching the students. I might as well have been a mannequin! I was frustrated with him at one point. I was not an easy patient, I also kept interrupting his conversation with the students to ask questions. You can't fault me for that, it is my body after all. The procedure was quick, though during the procedure, I felt the pain of him cutting into my skin, and I screamed. Then the nurse gave me more meds (fentanyl). It felt like I was floating on air after that.

Post-procedure teaching was much emphasis on infection prevention, because the catheter is threaded through the major artery resting close to the base of my heart. The right side of my neck felt numb, and I had pain on my right upper chest, a few inches below the clavicle (site of the port).

1st Chemo
July 9

> I love the Lord, because He has heard my voice and
> supplications. Because He has inclined His ear to me.
> Therefore I will call upon Him as long as I live.
>
> —Psalm 116

I slept very little last night. I was concerned about dislodging the port. I can feel the catheter on my neck. I hope it gets better with time. I took my prechemo meds; I hope I can keep track of it. Some I must take a day before chemo, some the day of, and few days after the treatment, then I get a break for about two weeks, and the circle starts again the third week.

I met with Dr. Goel, and she went over the medications and what to expect with me again, also informed me I would need to get a brain CT scan. *Just when I thought I was done with all the scans!*

I had a good corner by the window, Veronica and Tabatha were with me, they prayed with me as the first infusion started at about 11:30 a.m. The nurse was nice; she informed me that the first day is the longest because they infuse the meds very slowly. She kept a close eye on me, asking me every now and then how I was feeling. I did not feel anything; I thought I was going to feel the burning and all other strange effects, but nothing.

Got a visit from another friend from church who works there. She brought me some socks, I needed it. At my corner with all the girls, we had a good time talking and laughing. The day seemed to have flown by, and I received the last infusion at about 5:00 p.m. Got home feeling normal, I made myself some dinner and ate, waiting for the chemo effects to hit. Nothing! As I reflected on the day's happening—the chemo suite, faces I saw there today, the emotions of fear and sadness in some of those faces were so vivid to me—I whispered a prayer for them and for me, and I tried to get some sleep.

July 10

Still no side effects. I had my friend cut off all my hair today (I had it in braids). I did not want to wait for it to fall off. Although the doctor told me it will take two weeks from the first treatment for the hair to start falling off, I did not want to see chunks of hair falling out, so I chose to cut it very low.

July 11

Third day. Post-chemo, just a little tired. No serious fatigue, no nausea. However, I have not moved my bowels in three days. I have tried many things, drank more than half a bottle of laxative, yet nothing. It feels like my GI is closed for business!

July 12

> You, who have shown me great and severe troubles,
> shall revive me again, And bring me up again from the
> depths of the earth…and comfort me on every side."
>
> —Psalm 71

Feeling so sick today, very weak, lightheaded and dizzy, horrible taste in my mouth. I guess the effect has finally hit. I feel horrible!

July 15

The past three days has been very rough. Effects of chemo in full swing. Feeling very weak, dizzy, palpitations, horrible sore throat and sore tongue, bad heartburn, hardly slept, trying to make bowel movement sat on the toilet half the night, I feel lousy!

July 16

Mouth feels like lead. I juiced kale and celery today. Didn't taste half as bad as I thought it would be, but then I can hardly taste anything. I had a little more energy today. I was able to vacuum my room and change my bedsheets, and that made me feel good!

July 18

I was hoping to make it to church today but could not. I had a bad night. How I hate the taste in my mouth. My tongue feels so sore, terrible heartburn, I need a good night's sleep, and I feel miserable! Lord, I look to you!

Brain CT scan today (oncologist ordered). The technician was quite good-looking. I was embarrassed that he would realize that my beautiful hair was a wig! He was quite kind and offered me a cap because I had to take off the wig. I was made to lie on a hard steel table, then a dye injected into my veins, then he sets up the intimidating-looking CT scan swirling over my head. He instructed me not to move and then runs out the room, door closed behind him! Just me and the LORD now. I started meditating on Psalm 23 quietly, it brought me much peace and comfort.

July 24

Oh, Father, the journey is long, can I make it? I can see now that the road ahead is not going to be easy, the first chemo has taken a lot out of me, five more to go, Lord, I need you to carry me.

> When fear threatens to overwhelm you
> Take a deep breath and know He is your God
> When you feel like you are drowning
> Take a deep breath and remember God is in charge
> When you feel like you can't face another day
> Take a deep breath and remember He is ahead of your day
> When you are weak He is strong
> When you feel lost His eyes are on you
> When you have lost your fight
> Look to Him and get it back
> Do not give up
> God has everything under control!

Looking the Part
July 26

A few days ago, my scalp was so sore, I did not understand why, and in the shower this morning, I saw the rest of my hair washing off my head! And it was two weeks exactly after first chemo. It was a very emotional experience. I am bald!

I don't know why I am so weepy today, probably because I feel miserable with these flulike symptoms, annoying cough, and tightness in my chest. Although I have had incredible support from friends and families, I can't help feeling so alone today, and I am starting to look the part of a cancer patient with a shining bald head. Oh, Jesus, I trust you, hold me, carry me! Next chemo is Friday, please help me tolerate it well and reduce the annoying side effects.

I am bored already with these wigs!

July 28

My head feels like I am in a bubble half the time. Besides all the other symptoms, I was also not feeling good about myself at all, getting tired of the wigs, then at work, this lady comes in my office so bright and cheerful. "You look different," she said to me. "I like your hair, you look adorable." That lifted my spirit a bit.

Feeling better tonight, the tightness in my chest is relieved, the nasty cough is getting better, and I made some concoction of honey, ginger, lemon, and garlic and drank it all!

2nd Chemo
July 30

Treatment went well today. Tabatha was there to keep me company. I had a bad reaction in the beginning, severe pain in my pelvic area. The nurse stopped the infusions temporarily and gave me Benadryl. Afterwards, the rest of the day went smooth. I gave one of the patients there who was going through treatment for ovarian cancer a book by Pastor David Wilkerson *Have You Felt Like Giving Up Lately?* because she looked so sad and hopeless.

5

August 2

FEELING MISERABLE TODAY. Weak, mouth tastes horrible, nausea, and I have saliva bubbling up from my stomach I have to spit a lot. Four more cycle of these! Lord, I need grace.

August 8

A week after chemo, I feel much better. The bad taste in my mouth is getting better, no nausea, better appetite, I just cannot stand this rash in my face, however. Must be from the prechemo steroids.

My cousins flew in from ATL to be with me. So good to have them here to keep me company for a few days. Dieya is doing the cooking. I can get used to being spoilt like this!

My conversation with God
August 12

Lord, it's been a long time since I have gotten on my knees to pray. I feel like I am the weakest Christian alive. Although I have been strengthened by your presence, but physically it has been rough. Since May, it has been one assaults after another—all the barrage of tests, surgery, and now chemo. Sometimes, I wonder how much more my body can handle before it crashes. Father, I come tonight to draw near to you, not necessarily to ask for anything, but just to reconnect because I miss you! Lord, with all my frustrations and fears, you are all I've got. Hold me close, hold me close to your heart, and never let me go!

August 17

"I lift up mine eyes to the hills from where comes my help? My help comes from the Lord."

Feeling so alone today. The chemo effects are all in full swing. My period has stopped, and now I am getting hot flashes!

Had another inflation of my implant today at Dr. Samson's office by Samantha, the PA. I think it's almost as big as my right breast now, probably a few more to go.

3rd Chemo
August 20

My 3rd chemo went well today, I pray the side effects are minimal!

I was just thinking as I lay on my bed how loosely we use that word "I love you." During my time of crisis, seeing friends and families members rise up to the occasion has been truly amazing, even those far away who can't be here with me call me daily to see how I am feeling. How blessed I am! From the first day of chemo, I have not been alone in the infusion suite. My faithful friend Tabatha has been by my side like a rock, another friend readily available to cook and clean. My roommate, Veronica, going above and beyond, took time off work to accompany me to doctor visits, helping me with laundry, brings me food when I'm too tired to cook. To ensure I am looking good, our motto was "It's not how you feel, but how you look!"

I have also learned that talk is cheap; it is easy to say I love you and all other sweet words and yet not demonstrate it by actions. Don't call me from the comfort of your bed and tell me you love me when you have the means and ability to visit me. Love is not talk; it is an act. Show me love—don't talk it, demonstrate!

Lord, help me to be one that shows love by my actions. I know I do not have that ability to be what I should be, but I know I can do all things through Christ who strengthens me. Father, bless my dear friends and families, you know everyone and every sacrifice that each has made, reward them generously for their love. Amen.

August 24

These few days has been very tough—palpitations, aches, and pain. The worst of all—GI symptoms; my tongue is as white as chalk, and it feels like lead. Food has no taste, constipation that nothing seems to help, acid reflux, and the list goes on and on! I have not had a good night's sleep for days; the hot flashes, coming with more intensity and frequency, keep me up at night. One minute I am cold, next I am hot with profuse sweating! The sleeping pill the oncologist prescribed is not doing much for me. I feel lightheaded, my eyes are teary nonstop; it is so embarrassing. I thought third time around would be easier; the opposite is true. It seems like the side effects are more intense and lingering longer. This feels like the breaking point! Three more to go, I can't wait for the last treatment. Oh, Father, help me to finish!

August 30

Since I started chemo, I have been craving all sorts of food. Things I usually don't eat and some fruits and vegetable I normally couldn't tolerate in the past, I'm now eating them. Mangoes and pineapple is a staple around the apt, I just have to have them. Also bought a juicer, I have been juicing fruits and vegetables. A friend from church also gave me some barley powder, need to get more. I truly feel these fresh fruits and vegetables are helping me with my energy level and also helping with my blood count, which, although low, but not dangerously low.

6

September 5

LOOKING AT MYSELF today in mirror, it was a very strange feeling. The face looking back at me in the mirror looked so sick—bald head, swollen eyelids, red and teary eyes, it felt like that face belongs to someone else, because I certainly did not feel like that. At that moment, I felt somewhat strong on the inside.

When God is Holding Your Hand

When God is holding your hand,
There is peace that passes all understanding,
There is strength in weakness,
There is joy in sickness,
There is hope for tomorrow,
When God is holding your hand!

4th Chemo
September 10

Two more to go! Now, I have to wait for the effect to hit! I hope it's not a big one like last time.

> Hear O Lord when I cry with my voice: have
> mercy also upon me and answer me.
>
> —Psalm 27:7

September 11

Good day…Moved my bowel twice!

September 14

I had a bad night, long day at work, flulike symptoms, mouth tastes horrible, I should have taken the day off!

September 25

I have had a good few days, thank God! My energy level has been pretty good all week. I have not taken my iron pills since last chemo. I wanted to experiment, to hold off on the iron, because of the constipating effect and just take barley, beets, and carrots juice until my next blood test to see what the level would be. Not sure if it is a wise thing to do. I am not taking laxatives anymore; it contributes so much to the horrible taste in my mouth. Will try natural stuff and stool softener.

7

5th Chemo
October 1

ONE MORE TO go! My blood count was in fair range, would have been better if I had continued with my iron. I guess it's back to the iron pills.

October 9

Having enjoyed relatively good health up until this cancer diagnosis, it is hard to realize that my system is compromised right now, and I must be careful with what I eat and how I prepare my food. I had a rude awakening this morning. I saved the chaff from the carrot juice in the refrigerator for two days, and I decided to bake carrot cake with it. I baked the cake yesterday evening. It was so good that I ate so much of it! I woke up at about 6:00 a.m. this morning with a terrible stomachache; I ran to the toilet. I was nauseous, had diarrhea, diaphoretic, chills, and I was about blacking out. I seriously thought I was dying. Not wanting to be found dead alone, I quickly ran out the bathroom, banged on my roommate's door, and ran back to the toilet. She came out, prayed for me, good to have another nurse around at times like this; she guessed it was food poisoning. Just as quickly as the onset of symptom, so was the relief. After a little while on the toilet, I felt much better.

A week after the 5th chemo, seems like the GI symptom is taking longer—heart burn, constipation, bad taste in my mouth. I can't wait to be myself again!

October 15

Just to think a week from today I would have had my last chemo! I pray radiation would be a breeze.

The past week has been uneventful, 2nd week post-chemo, I feel pretty good, occasional fatigue at the end of the day. The GI symptom is minimal now; appetite is ravenous. I feel like I am losing control, I am eating everything and anything in sight, must be the steroids! I need to watch myself before I blow up.

October 17

"So the Lord blessed Job in the second half of his life even more than the beginning" (Job 42:12).

October 18

God has been so gracious to me at work. The office staff has been so helpful and caring. Most of the students with chronic illness requiring more of my attention has transferred to another school. My daily walk-ins are few—in fact, traffic to the medical room is very minimal. God knows I have but little strength right now. I actually have time to make my tea and time to nap during my lunch break! *Lord, thank you for taking such good care of me.* Four more days to my last chemo!

October 22

I can't believe that it is over, last chemo today, woo-hoo! I know I still have nine months of Herceptin to go; however, it does not have the hash side effects like the two chemos. It feels like these few months flew by. I can't wait to be myself again. Lord, I need a miracle tonight—a good night's sleep!

October 28

Almost a week post-chemo, my mouth still feels like lead. I haven't had a good night for a week. Sleeping pills are not helping, and my body feels like a ticking clock. Lord, help!

Next Stop, Radiation
October 29

Had a follow-up appointment with Dr. Rosenbaum Smith today. While in the waiting area, I could not help observing some anxious faces in the room. It brought me back to that frightful week of my cancer diagnosis; I know so well what they are going through. Selfish though it is, I was so grateful to have already gone through what they are probably anticipating; it felt so good to be on the other side! It was good to see the doctor again, and she was very pleased with my progress.

From there, I went to see Dr. Andrew Evans, radiation oncologist, and his team at the same institution, I was first seen by the nurse practitioner and then the oncologist, who thoroughly explain what radiation and treatment entails. Then it was off to the treatment room where I met with the radiation technicians. The radiation machine looked very intimidating! The area to be treated was marked ("tattooed") with permanent black markers. CT scan and X-rays were done on the areas to be radiated as part of the preliminary phase. Then I was custom fitted (molded) to be used for positioning during treatment. I was told treatment would be Monday through Friday for five and a half weeks, which would be a challenge to drive into the city daily after work for that time period!

8

November 3

I THINK I can see some fuzz on my scalp! Could my hair be growing back so soon, not even a month since my last chemo? I am still very fatigued though, I feel like an old lady—every bone in my body hurts, especially the hip area.

November 11

It was good to go in for Herceptin treatment today for just 30 minutes and not the whole day!

November 15

Practice run today for the radiation treatment. The nurses and technicians were all very friendly and encouraging. I was instructed to lie on my back on the uncomfortable treatment table surrounded by the intimidating machines. I was required to lie very still. The most unnerving moment was when they all hurried out of the room and watching the steel door close behind them! Got a few zaps of X-rays to prepare for the procedure starting next day. After the procedure, I was overwhelmed, and I cried; I just didn't feel like being strong at that very moment, so I gave in to my exhaustion and allowed my tears to flow freely as I drove home.

> My help comes from the Lord who made
> the heavens and the earth. The Lord stands
> beside you as a protective shade

—Psalm 91:4

> The Lord keeps watch over you as you
> come and go both now and forever.

—Psalm 121

November 16

The first radiation treatment went without a hitch. I was made to strip from my waist up then laid on my back on the molded material placed on the bed. I was positioned by the techs then instructed to keep very still as they hurried out of the room with the vault door closing behind them. The machine remotely controlled by the technicians zaps me in all the various areas that was tattooed. I was surprised because I was expecting to feel something. Surprisingly, I felt nothing during the treatment nor did I see the red beams I imagined (like you see in the movies)! I did not see or feel anything, just a buzzing and clicking sound. The treatment took less than 5 minutes.

November 18

I could not understand why I felt so nauseous all day. Was it the radiation or side effect of the Herceptin? Regardless, I refused to take the anti-nausea pills from the chemo treatment; I just did not want anything to remind me of the chemo, so I endured the nauseous feeling rather than take the medication!

November 27

Roughly two weeks of radiation treatment, and it seems to be going smoothly, although sometimes it is annoying to get there only to find out that the machine was broken or they had a special procedure and would have to wait longer than anticipated. I am so thankful that I have been able to find meter parking each day without any trouble. Even with the meter expiring before I get there, I have not gotten a ticket yet!

9

December 4

THIRD WEEK OF radiation. The technicians and the nurses has been so kind to me.

> I lie awake thinking of you, meditating on you through the night. I think how much you have helped me; I sing for joy in the shadow of your protecting wings. I follow close behind you, your strong right hand holds me securely.

> —Psalm 63:6–8

December 8

Radiation has been very frustrating these few days. Scheduling has been so unpredictable, was even cancelled without notice. I just can't wait until this ordeal is over!

December 10

Had a scare today as I went in for my follow-up mamo and sono on the only breast I had left. After the mamo, I was made to wait while the physician looked over the films. It seems to be taking too long; it was nerve-racking! Then off to sono. I had to wait a while also after the procedure because the doctor had to look over the films. I was finally told it was ok to leave. *Oh, Lord, I hope there is nothing wrong with my only breast!* Got the result at last. Everything is fine!

December 17

Radiation was uneventful this week. Almost the end of the week and things has been very smooth, thank God!

December 22

Waiting for my turn to get zapped at the radiation unit, and as various patients come in and out most used to the routines, some even cracking jokes with the nurses and technicians, it felt like I was part of a new community consisting of the radiation nurses, technicians, doctors, and the patients. I couldn't help but reminisce about the first time I received that dreadful news of cancer, the horror that accompanied the news, and now with surgery and chemo behind me, and now getting accustom to the daily radiation routine. As I observed the relaxed attitude of most patients and staff, I wondered what it must have been like for each of these patients the first day they received their dreadful cancer diagnosis too. The power of human resilience is amazing—as one passes through the various phase of life with its twist and turns, growing, changing, and adapting through each phase.

I feel a sense of sadness at the thought of not seeing these people I have met along the way again after my treatment. Truly, God has walked with me every step of this journey; even the bitter he has made sweet. I don't know what I would have done without Him!

December 29

I had a nice break from radiation, was allowed to miss a few days to go be with my loved ones for Christmas. I had a happy Christmas, I couldn't have asked for a better one! I came back to a snow-covered city. My car completely buried, it's going to be a challenge getting to radiation with the train and bus. I am at the point of exhaustion at this point. My radiated area is totally black. I wonder if it will ever be back to normal. The doctor seems to be satisfied with the way it looks; I hope he knows what he is doing! Two more zaps, and I am free!

December 31

This past year has been quite a year like no other, yet, Lord, just as you promised, you have been there with me every step of the way. You kept me from dismay, you held me up by your righteous right hand, you took away my fear and replaced it with peace, you were by my side during surgery, chemo, and radiation, you strengthened me in my darkest night. Father, you have been so faithful to me, you brought me through with blessings on every side, even my finances have not diminished with so much copays I can barely keep track of. I have more and not less; You have prospered me through it all. With just 50 minutes left of 2010, I want to thank you with all my heart for your goodness and faithfulness to me, for all you have done, and all you are going to do. Thank you, Lord!

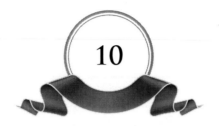

10

January 3, 2011

LAST RADIATION. Do I hear some cheers! I am so totally exhausted. I have this general feeling of achiness from my neck to my toes; I just want to be in bed for days on end! I cannot wait to be myself again.

January 4

"I am holding you by your right hand, I the Lord your God. And I say to you, do not be afraid I am here to help you...I am the holy one of Israel" (Isaiah 41:13).

January 9

I hope my body bounces back soon. I have been so fatigued these few days. Generalized achiness especially at my joints, still getting hot flashes—though with less intensity and less frequency—stomach feeling gassy, I have no energy. My laundry is piling up, almost out of towels, no energy to go to church today, looking forward to feeling normal again.

January 12

I am beginning to get frustrated. It is almost two weeks since my last radiation, and instead of feeling better, it seems I am getting worse. Besides the generalized achiness, I feel so fatigued, spent most of the day on the sofa today and still not feeling rested. I am concerned about where I'll get the strength to go to work in the morning. Took some meds for pain last night, didn't seem to work much. Took two Motrin tonight, I hope it relieves the pain, and I get a restful night.

January 13

I voiced my concern regarding the aches and pain and fatigue to the oncologist and was told it is a normal process and to give myself a few months to recover. Months! I was expecting to be back to myself immediately after radiation, but instead, I feel like a 90-year-old woman; it takes me a few minutes to get up from the sofa!

11

February 2

ONE MONTH postradiation. The skin that was so black has peeled off, and the area looks like my normal color, only a little lighter. It is a little over three months post-chemo. My hair is growing back, it's like baby hair—very straight and fine, the back seems thicker than the front, a little disappointed because the grey is back! I was hoping for a jet-black color. Also, it just dawn on me that I haven't had any hot flashes for a few days. The difficulty of sleeping still persists though.

February 4

Herceptin went well today, just 30 minutes infusion. And from there, went to see the plastic surgeon. He says I need more inflation to stretch the skin because the radiation has damaged and caused the skin to tighten.

February 19

I do not remember when I stopped having the hot flashes. I just realized it was not happening that frequent anymore, and now it has stopped. My hair is growing back, although I won't say I am ready to climb a mountain, however. I am not as fatigued as I used to be.

March 19

My period came back today. Welcome back, Anne flow!

April 6

Had flulike symptoms (fever and cough) for a few days that was not going away. I called the oncologist, Dr. Goel, who advised me to go to the ER. I waited one more day, and the fever still persistent with coughing like I have never had before. I decided to go in to the ER Monday morning, was admitted (for two days) for pneumonia on the left lobe of my lungs (same side I was radiated). I believe the radiation has left my left lungs compromised. I got IV antibiotics and more pills to take home.

April 19

I am scheduled for my second phase reconstructive surgery tomorrow. Dr. Samson is going to remove the expander and replace it with the saline implant. He is also going to lift my right breast to match the left. I can't wait to have symmetrical breasts again or close to symmetrical. These few months, it has been a balancing act with the reconstructed breast up and the other down. Not sure how it will turn out as the skin has really taken a beating from the radiation. I pray all goes well tomorrow.

May 15

Had the permanent implant in. The right breast lift is beautiful! I wish the reconstructed breast was just as perfect, but I am happy with it. Dr. Samson and Samantha, his assistant, did an excellent job and have been so kind to me.

August 15

I had my last Herceptin treatment July 1st and prior to that, have been having this feeling of intense fatigue that grew worse after the last treatment. It lingered for about two weeks after treatment. Now, it is so good to feel like myself again. Went for a week vacation to see loved ones, had a relaxing time. Back two days ago, today had my port removed. So good to be free! Also had the nipple reconstruction. Can't wait to see the end product!

November 15

Had another surgery a few days ago on the right breast. It needed an added lift because the reconstructed side was still higher. Now they both looked balanced, although Dr. Samson warned me that gravity would eventually take its toll on the right breast.

I had a brain MRI today. On my follow-up visit to the radiation oncologist, Dr. Evans, I expressed my concern about the mild dizzy feeling I have been experiencing for a few weeks. He thinks it's nothing, but for my peace of mind, he gave me the choice of having a brain MRI done. I pray everything comes back benign.

November 28

I finally had the guts to call for the MRI result today. Normal findings, although I figured everything was fine when I did not get a call few days after. I wonder why the dizzy feeling. Probably chemo brain?

12

August 1, 2012

Wow, IT'S BEEN over two years since the diagnosis and treatment. It seems like yesterday, a year since my last Herceptin treatment. I like my post-chemo hair—softer texture curls, don't need to perm it any longer. I have decided to keep it natural for now. I have been experimenting with various natural hair products; I might even open my own line of natural hair care product one day!

Also, for skin care, I have switched to natural products. I read labels a lot these days, and it is amazing how much chemicals are in the products we use day-to-day. I try to avoid cosmetics and products with phthalates and parabens in it, as I read that phthalates and parabens (methylparaben, propylparaben, etc.) can cause cancer.

My nutrition has changed drastically. I am more particular now about what I eat.

I gained almost 10 lbs. during chemo. I have lost 5, and I am happy with my current weight. People tell me I look even better now after cancer treatment! I still need to be more consistent with exercise for my overall good health.

Although I am not living daily in fear of the cancer coming back, it is a struggle, however, when I get sick with common ailments not to get anxious and thinking it might be cancer. I have been making frequent visits to my PMD lately. I hope he does not think I am a hypochondriac; I just don't take anything for granted anymore. I also still go on my scheduled follow-up appointments with the breast surgeon and the oncologist.

Sometimes, I get the feeling that people think I am a ticking time bomb ready to go off anytime; I am referring to the cancer coming back. It gets annoying when I have to constantly answer to the question, "The cancer is gone, right?" or "Are you ok? The cancer didn't come back right?" Yes, the cancer is gone, and, no, the cancer has not come back!

August 2014

Almost four years after my first breast reconstruction, I decided to go for a second reconstruction using my upper back skin and muscle (the latissimus dorsi) because the reconstructed breast was not so comfortable. The skin had been destroyed by the radiation, so the reconstruction was not very natural looking—it was very high in proportion to the other breast, it was hard, and the skin was tight. During one of my follow-up visits with Dr. Samson, I decided on redoing the reconstruction, and thankfully, I got the approval of my insurance. The procedure is called the *latissimus dorsi flap*. Initially, I thought he was going to cut a skin from my back and graft it to the left breast area. Little did I know the intricate process of the surgery, as he explained it to me. I also Googled the procedure and watched on YouTube. I cringed as I watched it. First, they cut an oval flap of skin, fat, muscle, and blood vessels from the upper back. This flap is moved through the skin under the armpit to the chest to reconstruct the breast. The blood vessels (arteries and veins) of the flap are left attached to their original blood supply in the back.

I went in for the first phase of the reconstruction. The damaged skin, which was predominantly in the lower half of my breast area, was removed, and the skin from the latissimus dorsi flap sutured to the upper breast skin, a new tissue expander also was put in to stretch the new skin. Post-op, I had two drains put in, one in my back and one on the breast area. I had fluids accumulating in the back area after the drain was removed. I was told that was one of the complications of the latissimus dorsi flap. I had to go back and forth to the doctor's office for about two weeks to have the fluids drained. Then about six weeks post-op, went in for inflation and periodically after that to stretch the skin.

April 30, 2015

My last inflation was early December, and then I was scheduled for the second phrase, which is the removal of the expander replaced with the permanent silicone implant. I had the exchange surgery in January. Feeling satisfied with the outcome, the skin is softer, and the implant looks and feels more natural. I had the nipple reconstruction at Dr. Samson's office a week ago. What a difference it makes. I feel like I have my breast back!

LIFE AFTER CANCER

I SUPPOSE ONE cannot help but see things differently after being faced with one's mortality. I am thankful to God for life, for health, and for the ability to work and earn a living. I am not too concerned about many things anymore. This is the fifth year of being cancer free, and with each passing day, the fear of recurrence becomes less and less, and I am more concerned with living for the moment. Life to me is a gift and very short; there is no need to add needless complication to it. I am happy and comfortable with who I am. I have more desire now to enjoy the simple things in life.

I am more cautious about what I eat these days; my nutrition consists mostly of whole foods, fresh vegetables, and fruits. Most of my fruits and vegetables, I buy organic. I also buy organic eggs and chicken, fish I try as much to get the wild caught rather than the conventional farm-raised ones; and when I do eat beef, I buy the organic grass-fed ones (not easy to come by though). According to a book I read (*The*

China Study), the grass-fed beef is rich in healthy omega 3, while the conventional beef is rich in omega 6. Omega 6 is said to increase the risk of inflammation and cancer and other autoimmune diseases.

It is funny how some people pass judgments without knowing the reason others do what they do. I remember the other time I was at a whole food supermarket, I was asking the guy in the meat department if they had organic grass-fed beef. I noticed the lady next to me rolling her eyes and muttering under her breath, "What's the big deal?" I was so tempted to answer her!

My favorite breakfast smoothie consists of organic kale, fresh pineapple, and a tablespoon of organic coconut oil. Sometimes I substitute coconut oil for low-fat organic yogurt. I particularly like drinking green smoothie in the morning because it so hard to get the necessary servings of vegetable each day, so starting my day with a serving or two makes me feel that I am doing something good for my body! I have cut down tremendously on sweets. I substitute sugar for agave because it is said to be low in glycemic index (does not raise the blood sugar as much as regular sugar). I have read from various sources that sugar feeds cancer cells, hence my trying to cut down on sugar/sweet consumption. I still need to be more consistent with my exercise routine. One day, I will get it together!

I feel deep compassion for those going through that dreaded word *cancer*, of course, having gone through it myself.

I have been having friends call me and asking if I can talk with someone they know that is going through what I have gone through. And each time, I gladly say yes because I remember when I was newly diagnosed, I just wanted to speak with someone who had gone through same thing. And thankfully, my friend Isi, who is a survivor herself, had a friend who had the same type of cancer I had and was successfully treated was my lifeline.

Each time I had questions, she was ever so helpful, and I was very encouraged by her, which is why I decided to put to print my personal journal.

I remember during my early treatment phase. I was working at another site for the summer as a school nurse. Ana, a lady I met there at summer school, was going through a very frustrating time with feelings of helplessness because her sister Lynn was also recently diagnosed with breast cancer. According to Ana, she didn't "know how to help" her. My coworker Diane told Ana about me, and she came to speak with me regarding her sister. As we talked, we realized that Lynn had a similar diagnosis, and what is more surprising, she was being treated at the same facility and by the same team of doctors as I was! What are the odds! So Ana was so happy, she linked me up with her sister, and since I was a few steps ahead of her in the treatment phase, I would tell her what to expect. We encouraged each other through the treatment process, and Lynn is doing great today.

My very good friend Isi, a young mother of one boy and twin girls, was diagnosed with breast cancer a few years before I was; the diagnosis came while she was nursing her beautiful twin girls. Little to say, we were all devastated and scared for her. Her focus at the time were her children, so she opted for mastectomy without reconstruction because according to her, she had neither time nor the energy for a protracted treatment; she just wanted to be home with her babies. About four years later, she was there for me during my cancer diagnosis; she watched me go through surgery, treatment, and reconstruction. She tells me later that I inspired her to go for reconstruction. So approximately five years after her mastectomy, she went for reconstruction, and she is doing great today with her beautiful family.

CONCLUSION

THROUGH THE WHOLE cancer ordeal, I have learned the importance of being proactive about one's health. Thanks to technology, there are no more excuses for anyone literate to be ignorant. There is a wealth of information available at our fingertips, and there is no excuse not to be informed.

Before the cancer diagnosis and the time of my going back and forth to Dr. T, I was very laid-back. I was content to listen to the doctor's recommendation because I trust he knew what he was doing. I did not do my own research, and although my breast was getting worse, I was very laid-back about it, and my laziness could have cost me my life. Seven years of being his patient, I did not request test results, and neither did I seek a second opinion until I had no choice but to do so. The three biopsies I had when under his care, all I heard him say was "benign," and I was satisfied. I was totally ignorant of breast pathologies and the fact that some benign breast disease does put one at risk for developing breast cancer; for instance, although all the conditions listed in my three biopsies with Dr. T were benign breast conditions, researchers suggest that hyperplasia with atypia and also sclerosing adenosis are all risk factors for developing future breast cancer. I also read that some of these benign conditions can co-occur with invasive cancer in the breast tissue, and I strongly believe that was my situation because an 8-cm DCIS and a 5-cm invasive cancer does not grow overnight.

I cannot overemphasize the importance of requesting copies of tests performed even if you don't understand what is written there. Be very proactive—it is your body, it is your life, know what your diagnosis is, read about it, ask questions, seek other professional opinion, go to a specialist in that field. In my case, Dr. T was a general surgeon who also performed breast surgeries. He was not a breast specialist. In fact, each time I went for my appointment with him, his office was packed with people for various surgical needs. I remember during one of those visits I was sitting on the examining table, and while he was looking over my sonogram result, he was dozing off right in front of me! Now, tell me how can a doctor who is so overworked with such an overload of patients be thorough with each patient?

I would also stress the importance of early detection. In breast cancer, survival increases with early detection and intervention; there is the temptation to adopt what I call a "head under the blanket" attitude of "I don't want to know." Well, what you don't know can kill you. Living in denial can do more harm than good. Instead of shying away from that overdue mammogram, take the bull by the horns and go for it. Because, again, early detection increases one's chance of survival.

My lackadaisical attitude could have cost me my life. My fear of cancer kept me from seeking answers in the earlier stages, and the cancer could have been in an advanced stage before it was diagnosed. I am thankful to the Lord that it was caught before it got too advanced, and I am also thankful for the excellent team of physicians, physician assistants, nurses, and technicians at Mount Sinai St. Luke's and Mount Sinai Roosevelt that helped put this humpty-dumpty back together.

Putting my personal cancer journey journal into print, I am hopeful that someone going through that dreadful diagnosis or a friend or relative can find encouragement and some helpful insight as to what lies ahead, although all treatments and outcomes are not the same; however, it is always good to hear a personal success story, and that encourages hope, because hope does not disappoint.

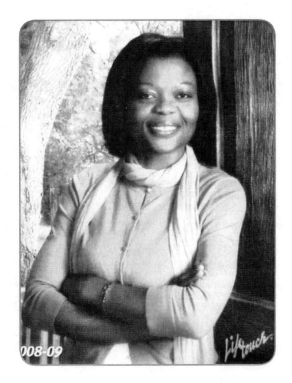

Before cancer diagnosis

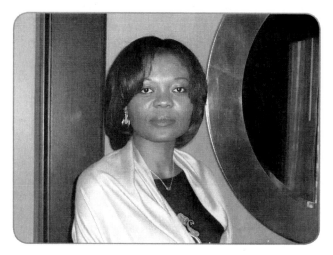

Shortly before diagnosis

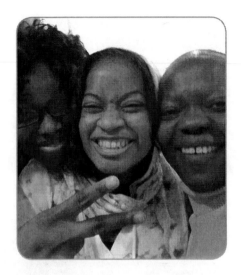

During chemotherapy

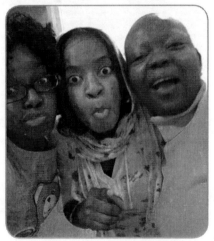

Selfie with Ese and Jennifer

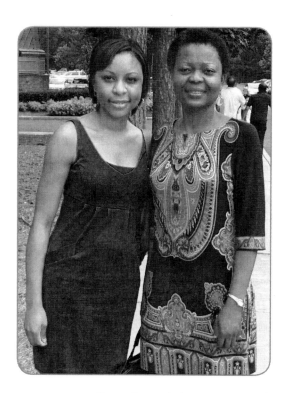

Post-chemo hair

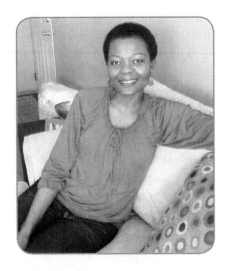

My hair growing back!

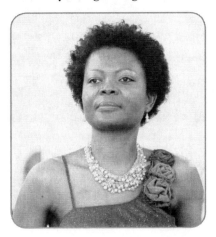

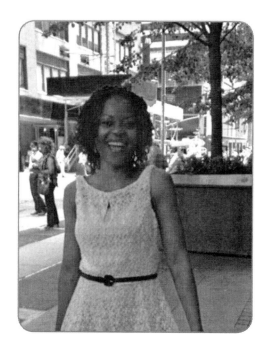

2013

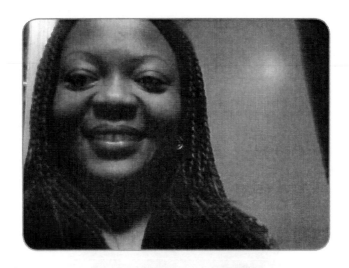

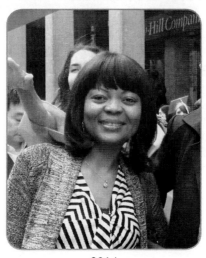

2014

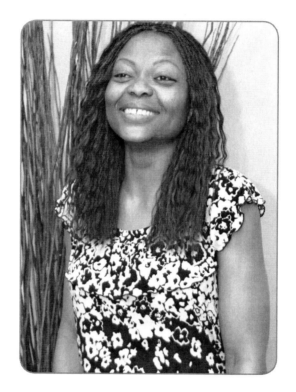

June 2015

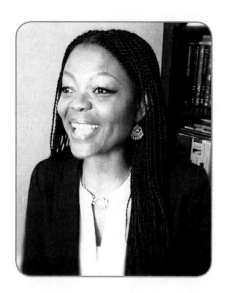

May 2015